Chubby's Tale

The true story of a teddy bear
who beat cancer

Written by Carola Schmidt
Illustrated by Vinicius Melo
Edited by Chris Roy

Second Edition
Fall 2021

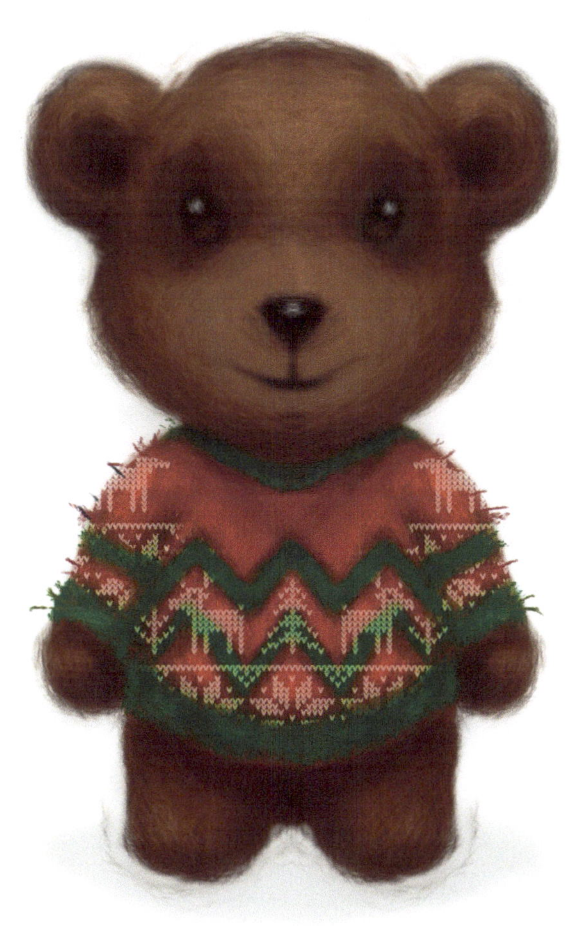

His tag says his name: Chubby.

He was a teddy bear with a wool pullover and no pants. He lived on a shelf in La La Land toy store. His dream was to be bought by a kid and taken to a real home.

Everything went well with Chubby's job. Sitting on the shelf, waiting for someone to come take him home. So the time passed smoothly since Chubby arrived at the store in a delivery truck. However, one day, things changed a bit. He felt unwell.

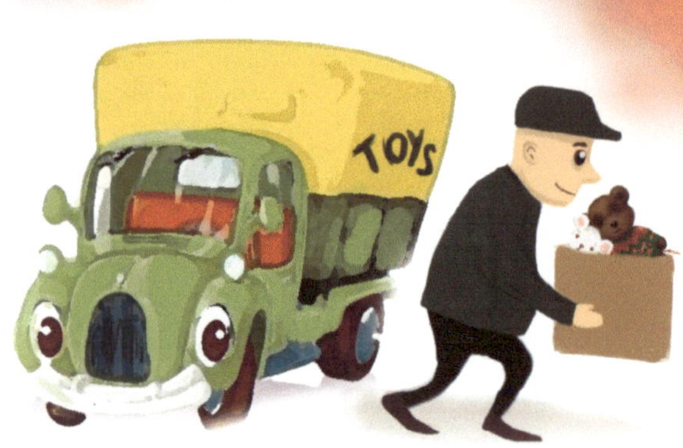

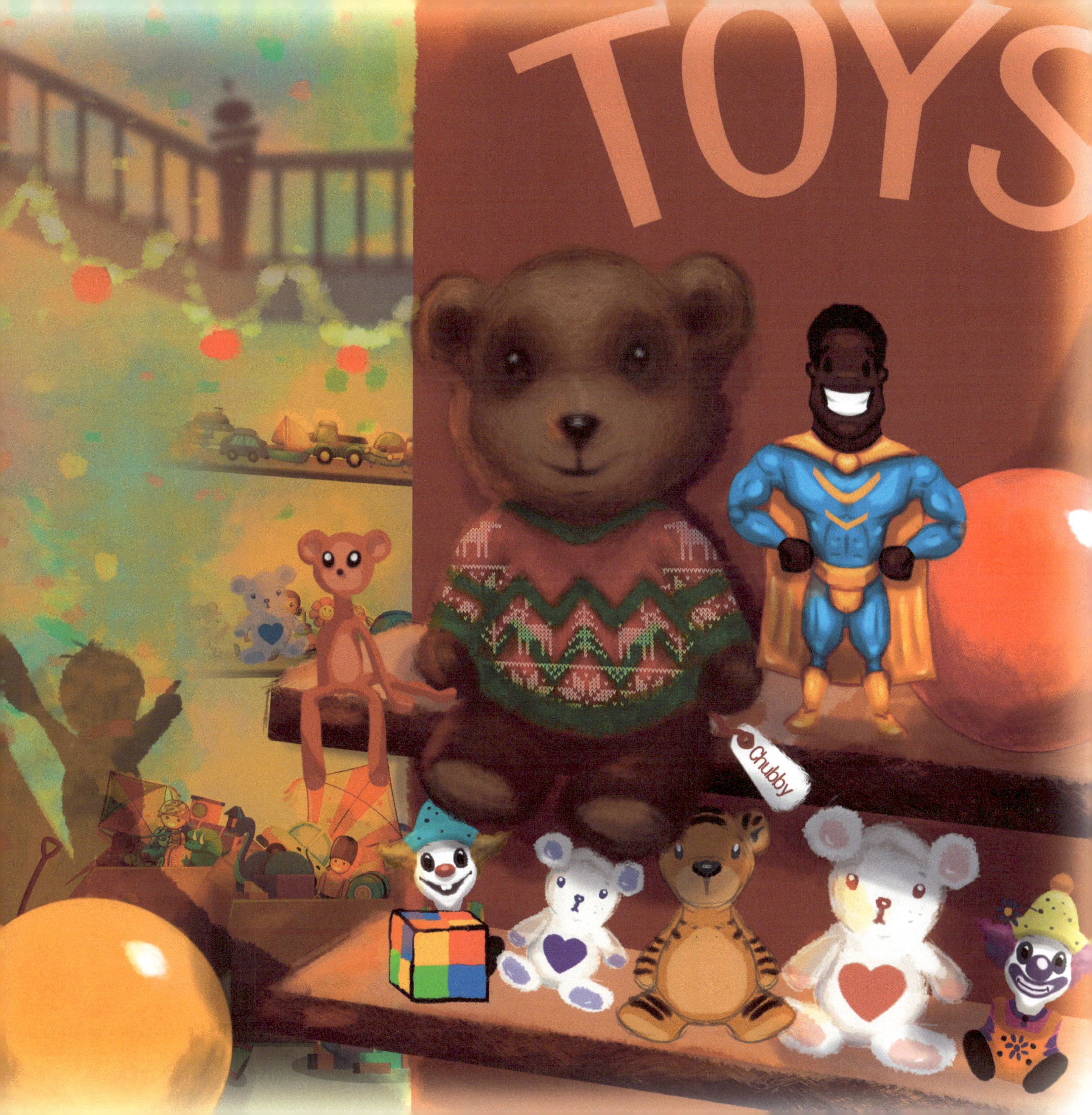

TOYS
Chubby

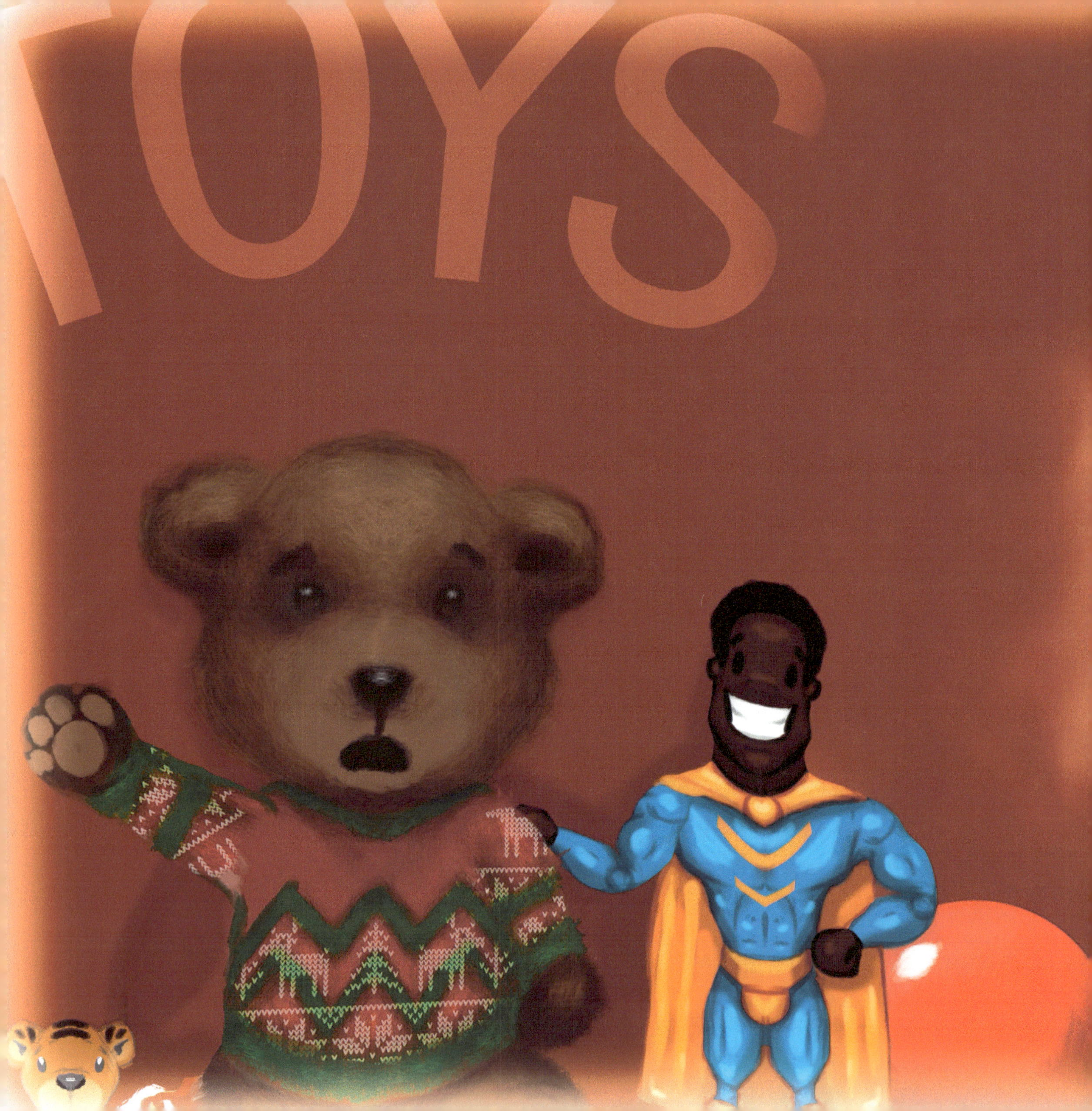
TOYS

"Are you OK, Chubby?" asked his shelf neighbor, Superhero.

"I don't know, Superhero. Maybe not."

"Oh man! Go find someone to help you get better. Christmas is around the corner. You know… Nobody buys toys after Christmas!"

"You're right, Superhero," said Chubby as he climbed down shelf by shelf until he reached the floor.

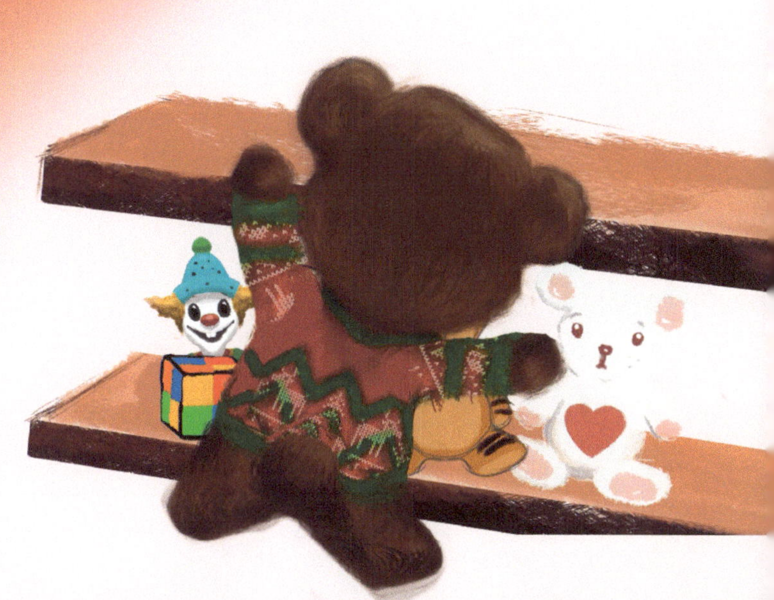

Chubby hurried to the elevator and pushed the button. Since the store was closed, the elevator arrived quickly. He pressed the button to the second floor. When the door opened again, Chubby saw a sign: Christmas Department. He had never left the first floor and didn't know that a toy store could have a Christmas department.

Maybe I'll find someone here that can help me, he thought.

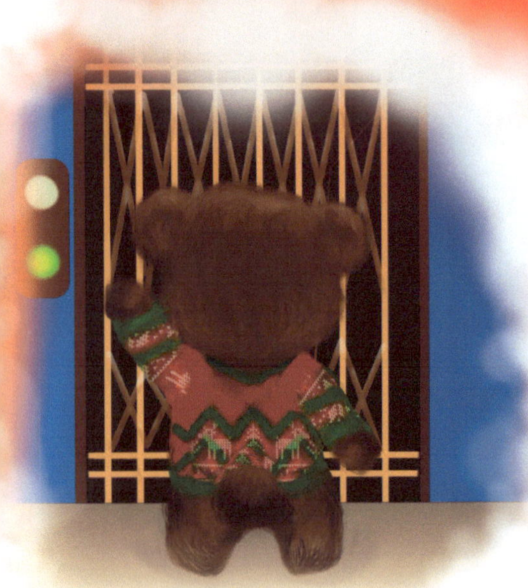

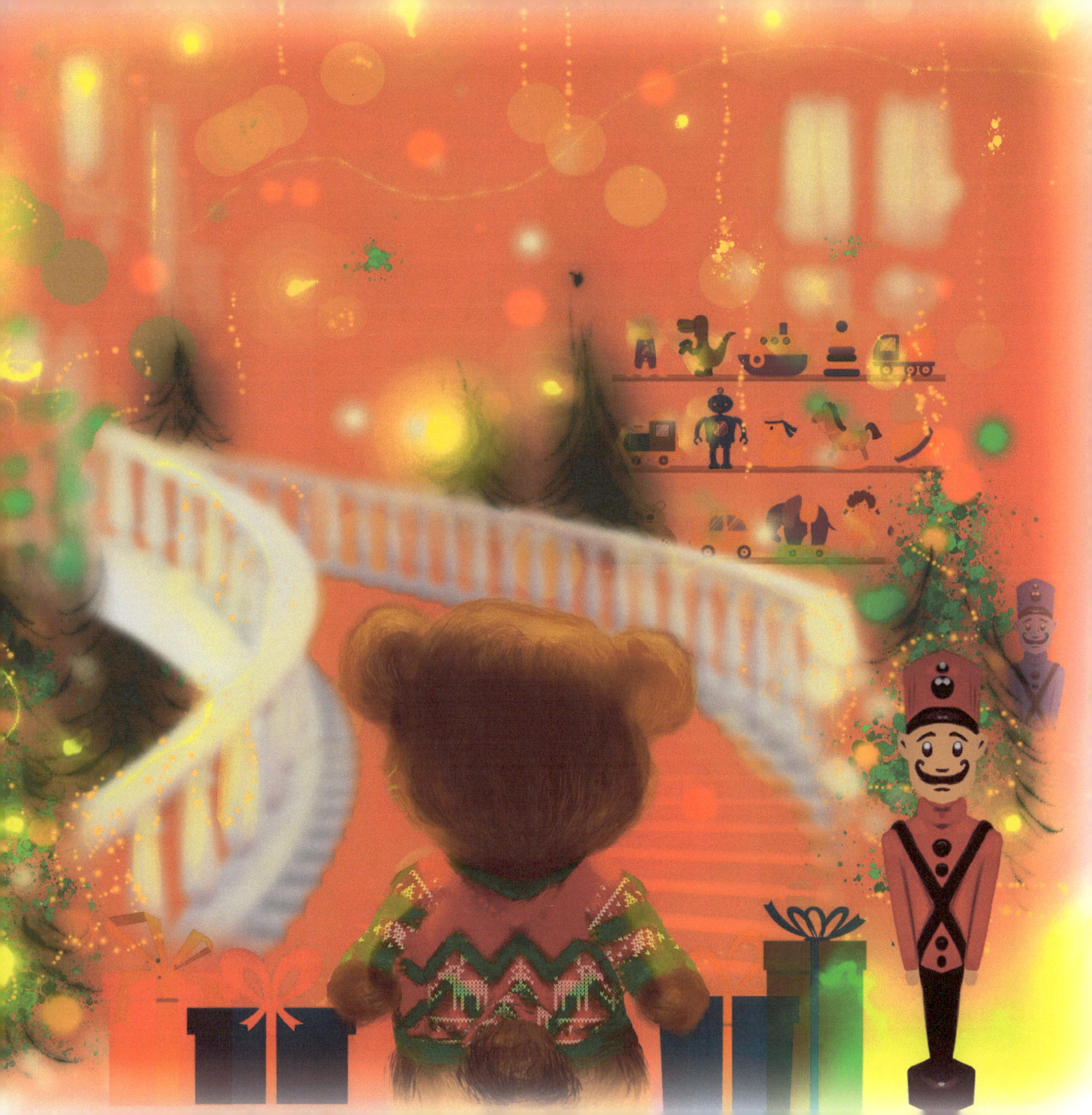

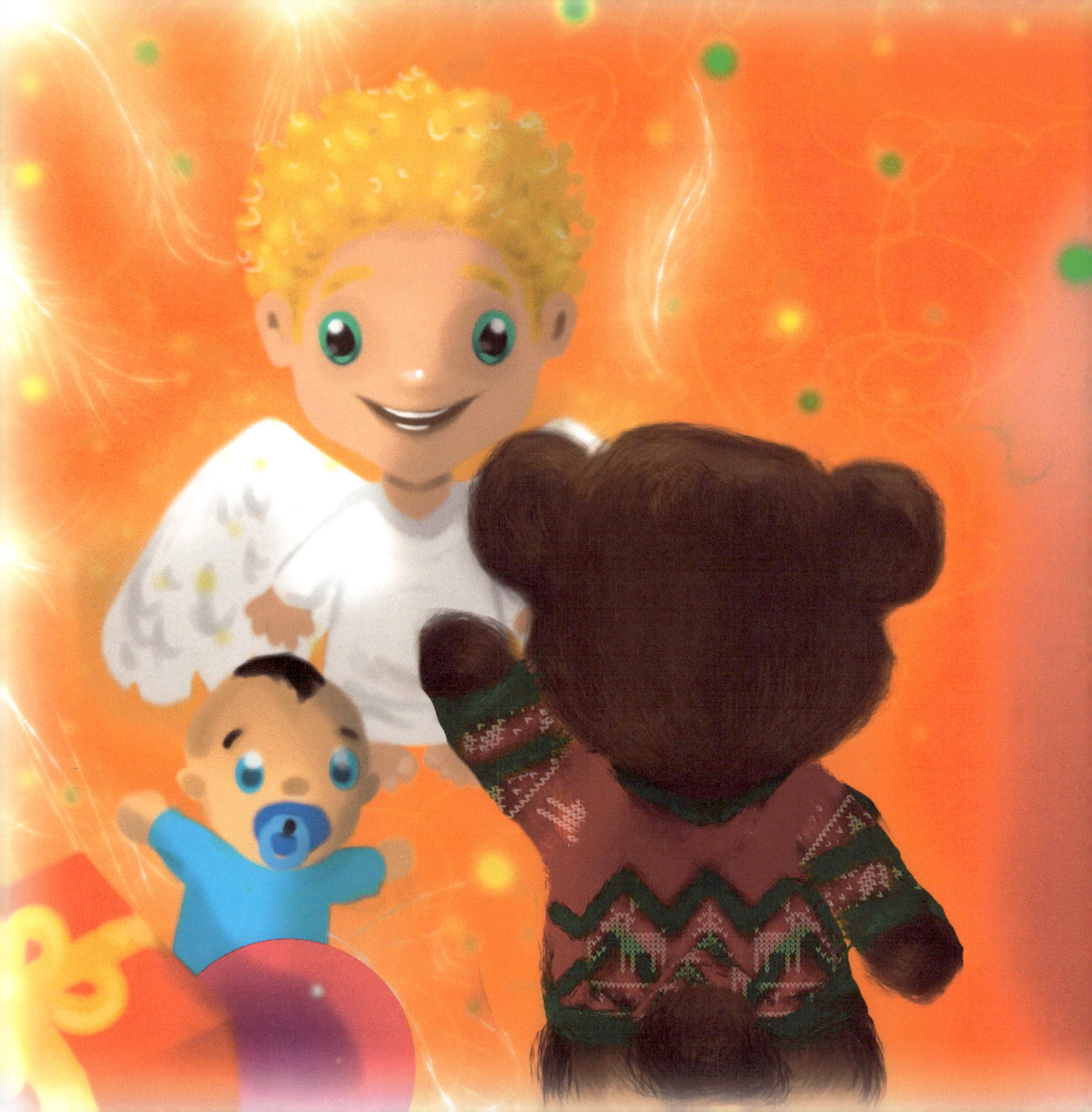

Chubby saw an angel with sparkling wings standing behind a little baby and went to talk to him. He said, "Guardian Angel, I don't feel well. Can you help me get better?"

"Yes, I can do it. I'll send you the cure. But you will have to find a doctor," the angel said. "Go to a doctor in the doll department! There is a collection of professionals, with doctors, pharmacists, nurses, ballerinas, scientists, and astronauts."

"Thank you, my Guardian Angel."

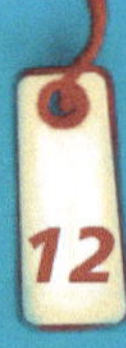

Chubby took the elevator again and went to the third floor. It was full of toy vehicles. There were trains, cars, drones, space rockets and countless other vehicles.

With a car, it'll be easier to find a doctor! Chubby thought, looking at the shelves.

"May I help you, sir?" a car dealer made of building blocks asked him.

"I'm looking for a doctor. I have to travel to the doll department so I need a car."

"To drive around the store… I think you might need a small car."

"You're right. Do you have an older model Beetle?"

"Yes, I have! Which color do you prefer?"

"Yellow."

"Great."

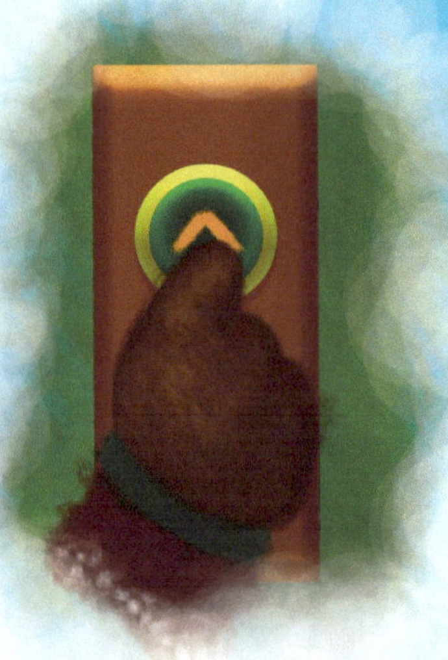

"I'll get some toy money and come back. Please, hold the yellow one for me," Chubby said.

"OK. I'll be waiting. There is toy money on the fifth floor."

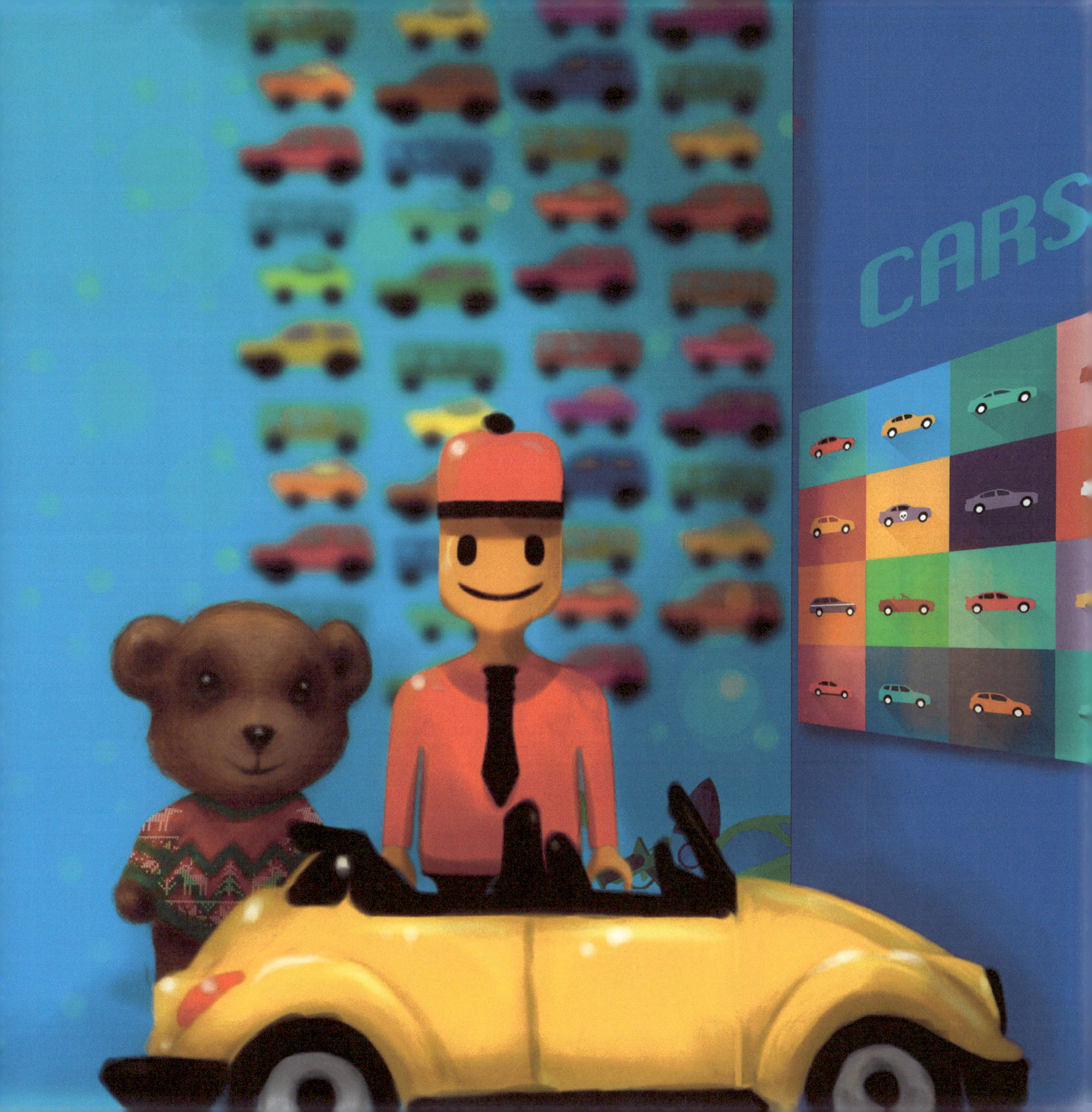
CARS

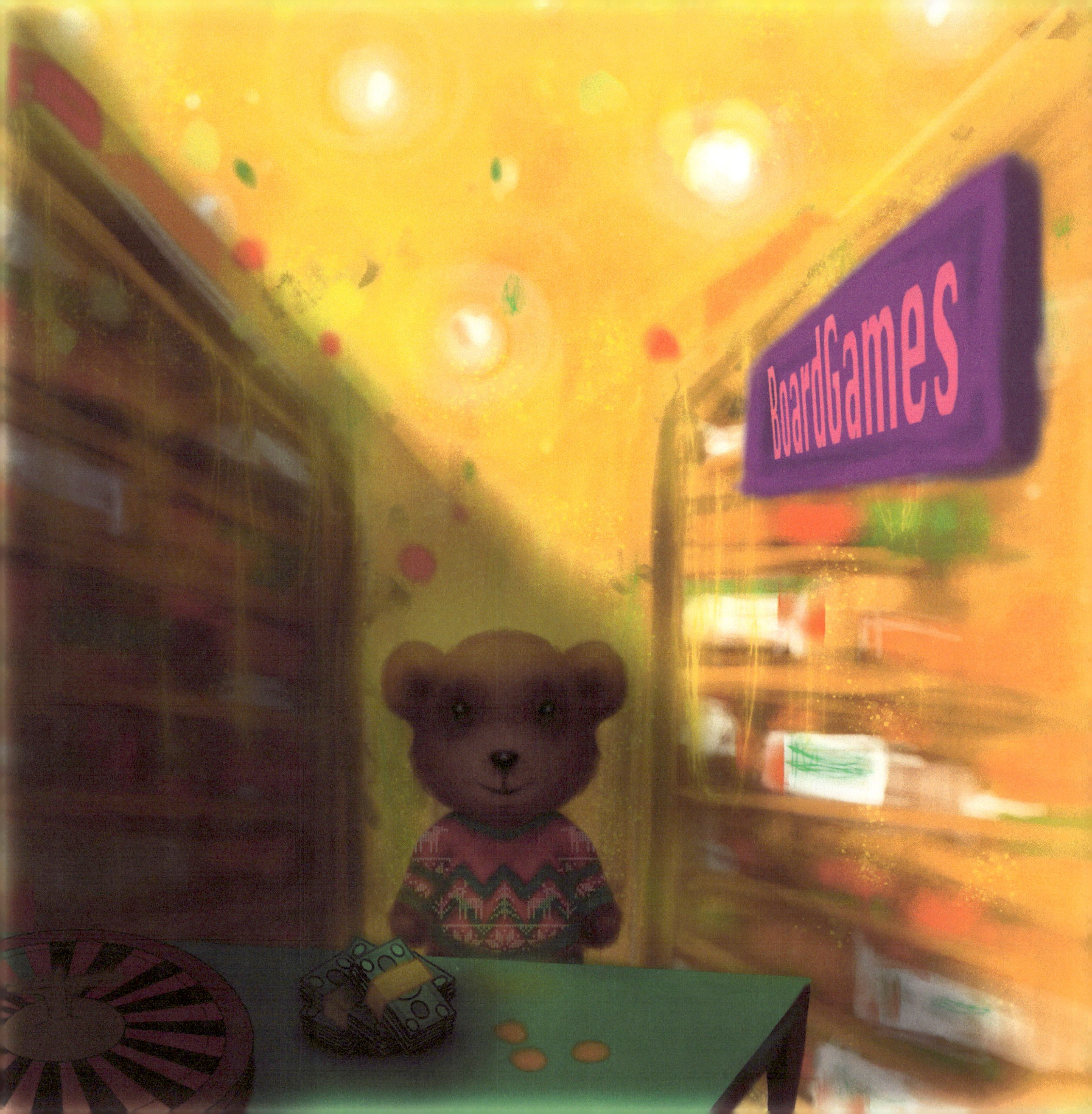
BoardGameS

Chubby took the elevator and went to the fifth floor and found the toy money quickly.

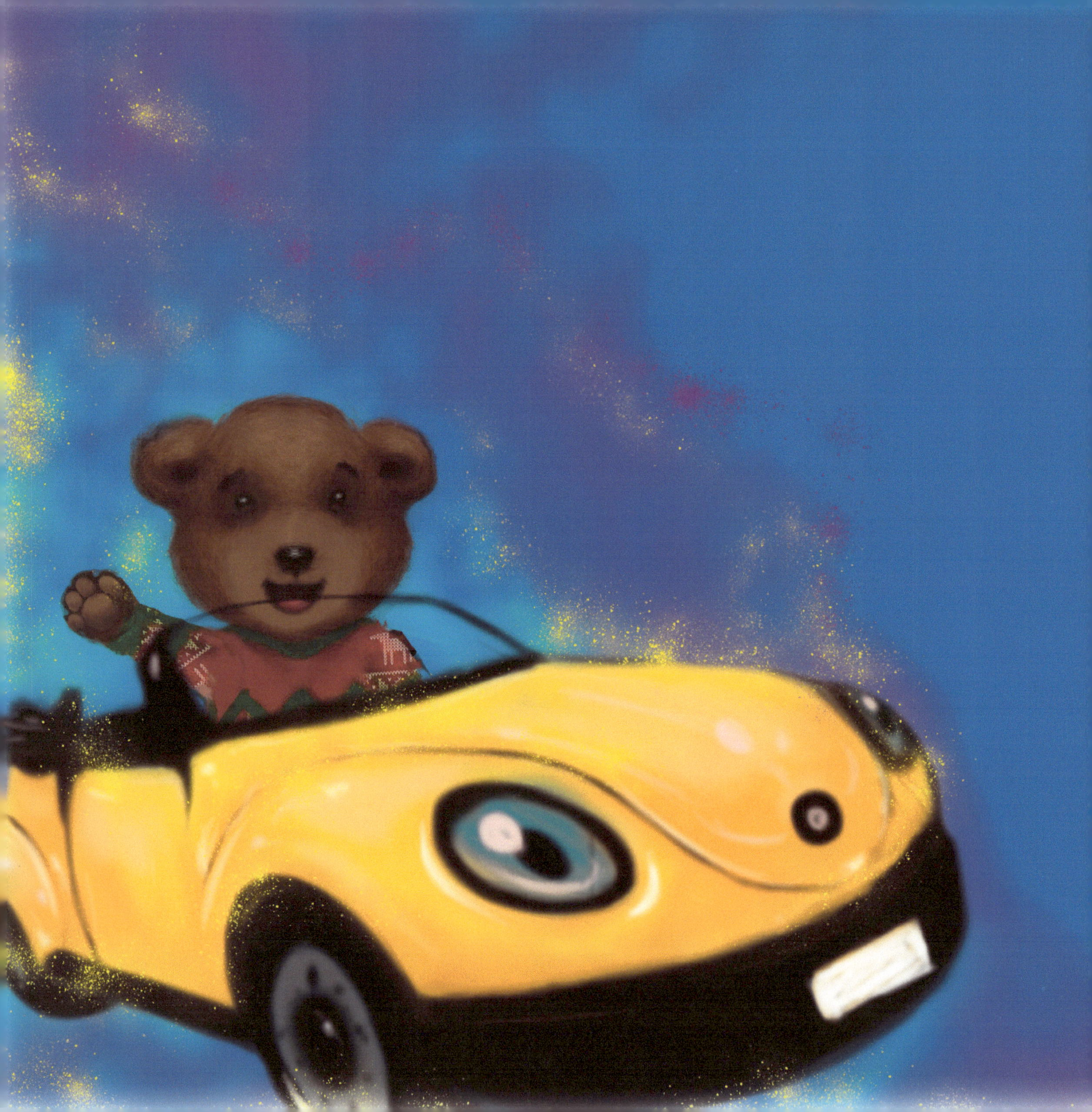

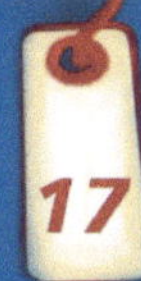

He went back to the third floor to get his car, a beautiful, yellow antique Beetle. *There is an advantage to having a new toy car*, he thought. *Even the old model is new!*

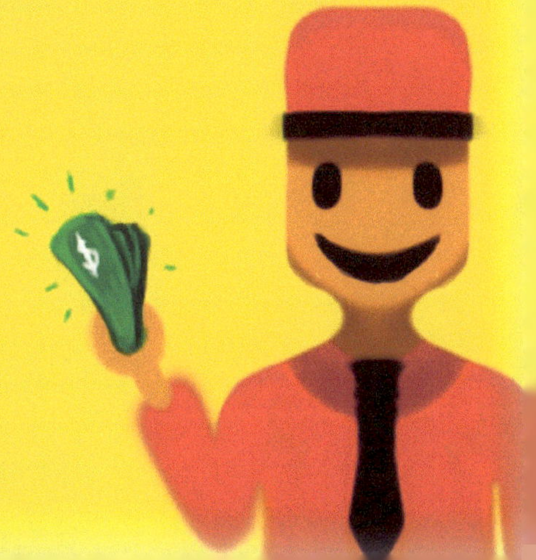

Chubby went back to the elevator, driving his car, to go to the sixth floor. As soon as the door opened, Chubby drove the Beetle out of the elevator and around the doll department to find a doctor.

"Doctor Doll," Chubby read on a box.

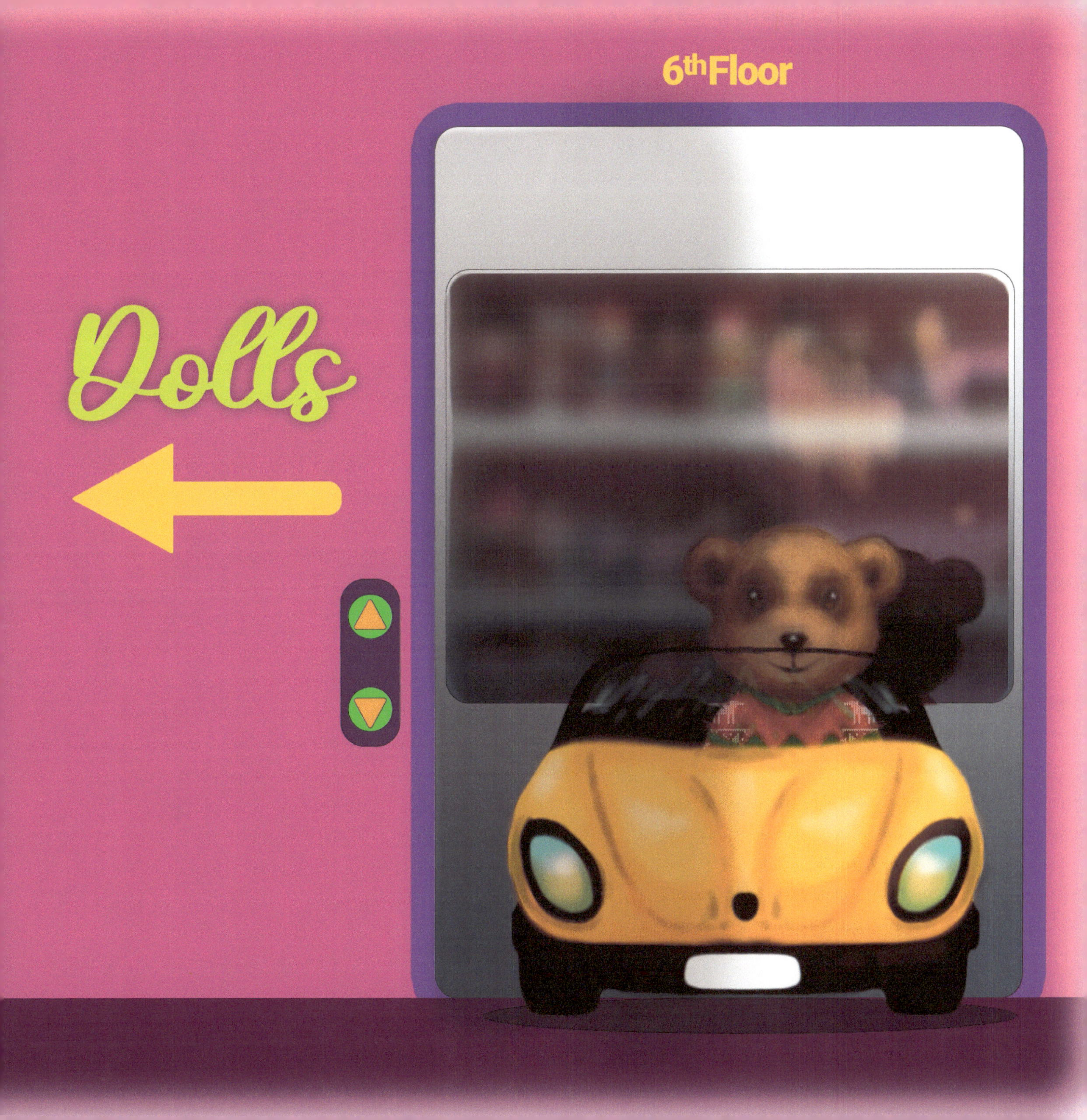

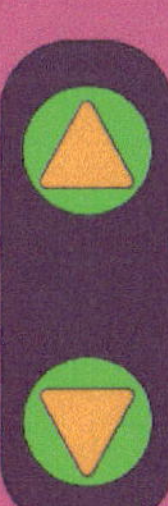

Dolls

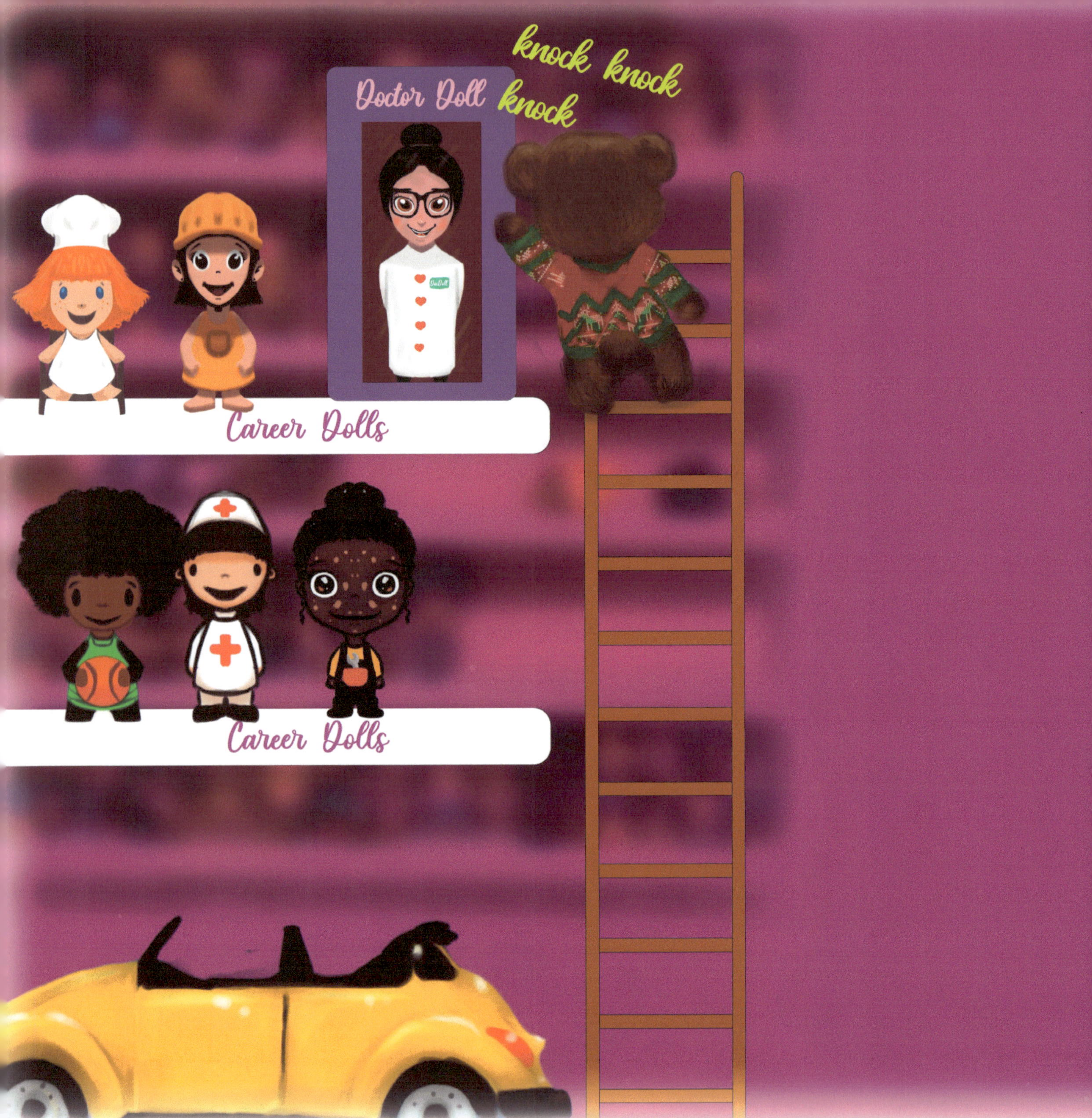
knock knock knock
Doctor Doll
Career Dolls
Career Dolls

After parking his Beetle, Chubby climbed up to the shelf where the doctor was displayed. He knocked three times on the box to call her.

"Please, open the box," Doctor Doll said, waking up.

"I'm sorry to bother you so late, Doc," Chubby said, opening the box.

"I'm glad you called me. I'm just stuck in this box, waiting for a kid. I was already bored," she said, leaving the box. "Tell me, what's your name?"

"Chubby. I don't feel well."

"OK, Chubby. We'll solve this." She began examining him.

"What do I have?"

"Chubby, you need to have some tests done. I'm going to use a very small needle and take a little drop of blood for analysis. My colleague is a specialist and will tell me exactly what you have. He's a scientist."

Chubby bravely said, "OK," already stretching his arm towards her. She took his blood.

"I'm proud of you, Chubby." She put the needle with his blood in a safe container.

"It didn't hurt at all, Doc." He looked at his arm and smiled.

Chubby was given a bed, a blanket and a pillow. He slept on the sixth floor, waiting for the blood test results. In the morning, the doctor woke him up.

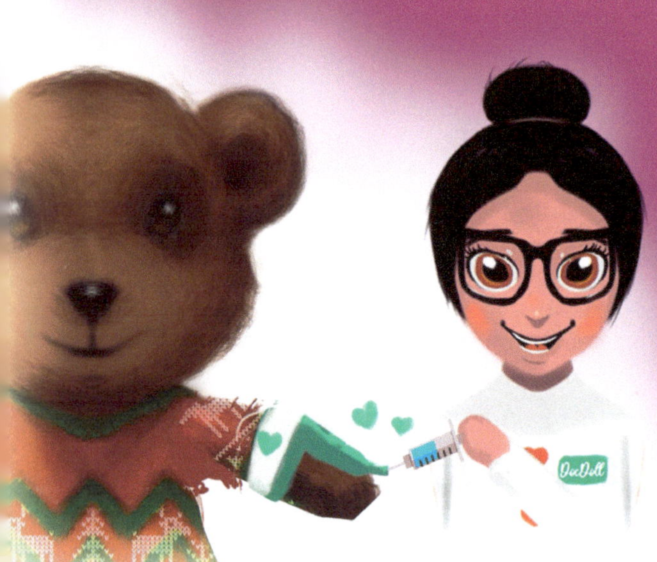

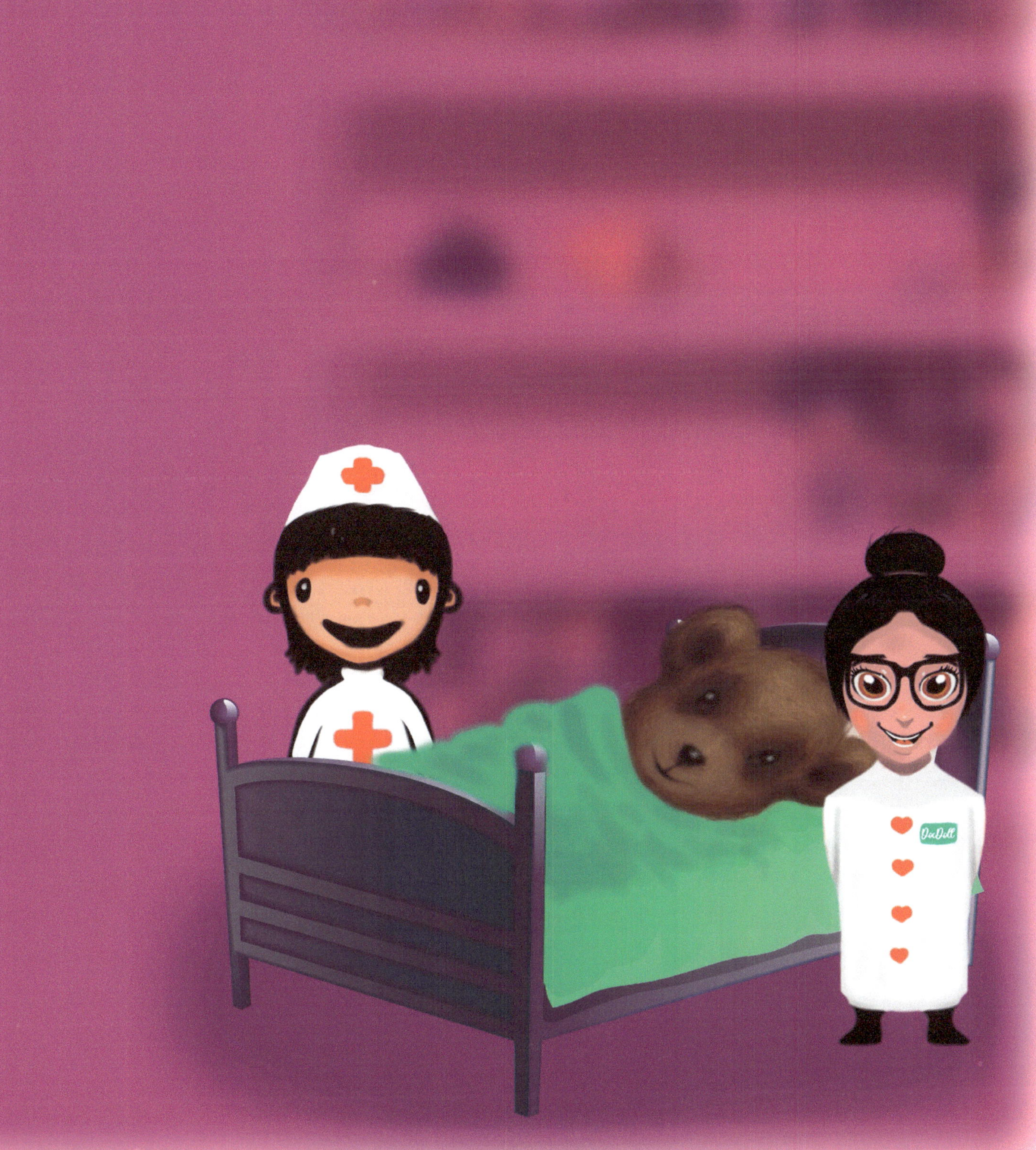

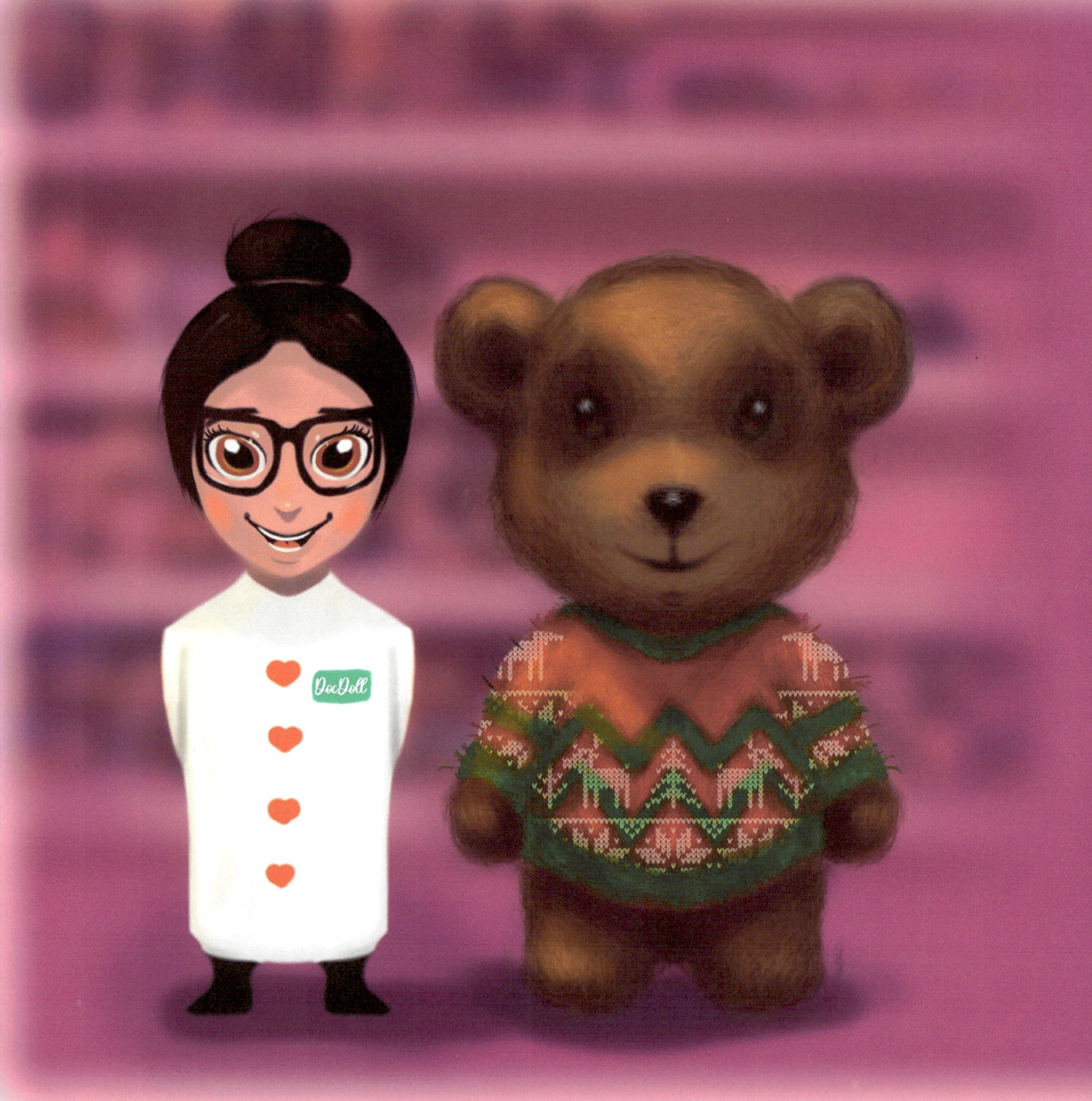
DocDoll

"Good morning, Chubby. We have your results."

"Good morning, Doctor Doll. What do I have?"

"You have an illness that we'll treat with chemotherapy, and you'll get better. The disease is called cancer."

"What is cancer?"

"Everyone is made of tiny cells. We cannot see them without a microscope, but together they form our bodies. There are many different types of cells in our bodies. Cancer occurs when a cell has a problem and becomes unhealthy. It becomes sick. The unhealthy cell creates more unhealthy cells. When someone has a lot of sick cells, we give them chemotherapy to heal them."

"OK," Chubby said thoughtfully.

"The type of cancer that you have is called leukemia. That means cancer in your blood. You have immune cells in your blood that protect your body against diseases. These immune cells are produced in a place called bone marrow. Your bone marrow is unhealthy and formed too many sick cells. We'll eliminate these sick cells with chemotherapy. But we also need to fix your bone marrow so it creates healthy cells. We will do this with stem cell transplantation."

"I think I understand. Stem cell transplantation will make my bone marrow healthy again, so it'll stop making sick cells, right?"

"Yes. First, you will receive chemotherapy to get rid of the unhealthy cells. Then we'll do a stem cell transplantation to fix your bone marrow. After this, you'll be healed!"

Patient: Chubby
Diagnosis: Acute Lymphoblastic Leukemia

It is the most common type of childhood and teddy bear cancer. It happens when bone marrow becomes sick. Bone marrow is a tissue inside large bones that makes blood cells. When bone marrow makes too many blood cells called lymphocytes, and they are not fully grown and don't work right, Acute Lymphoblastic Leukemia can develop.

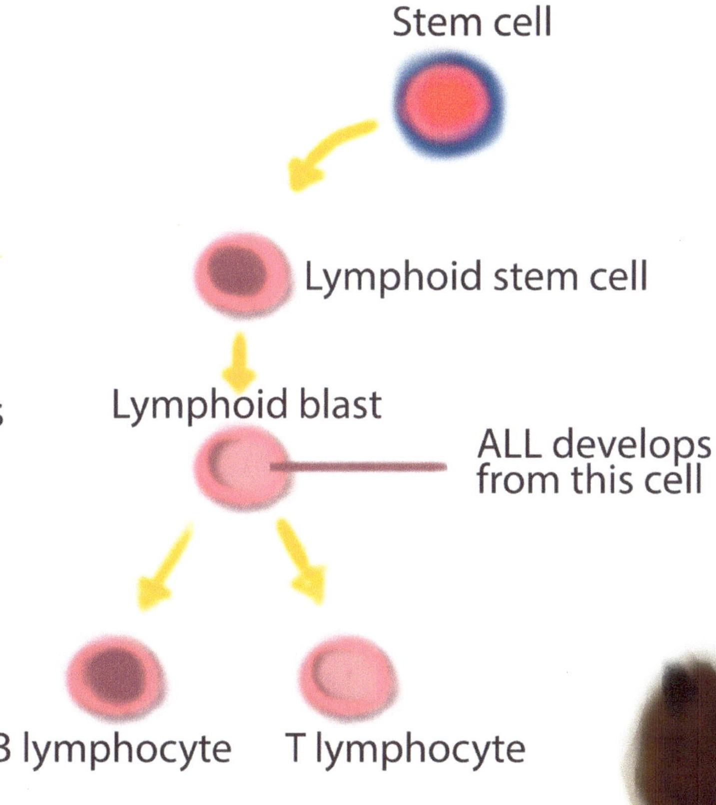

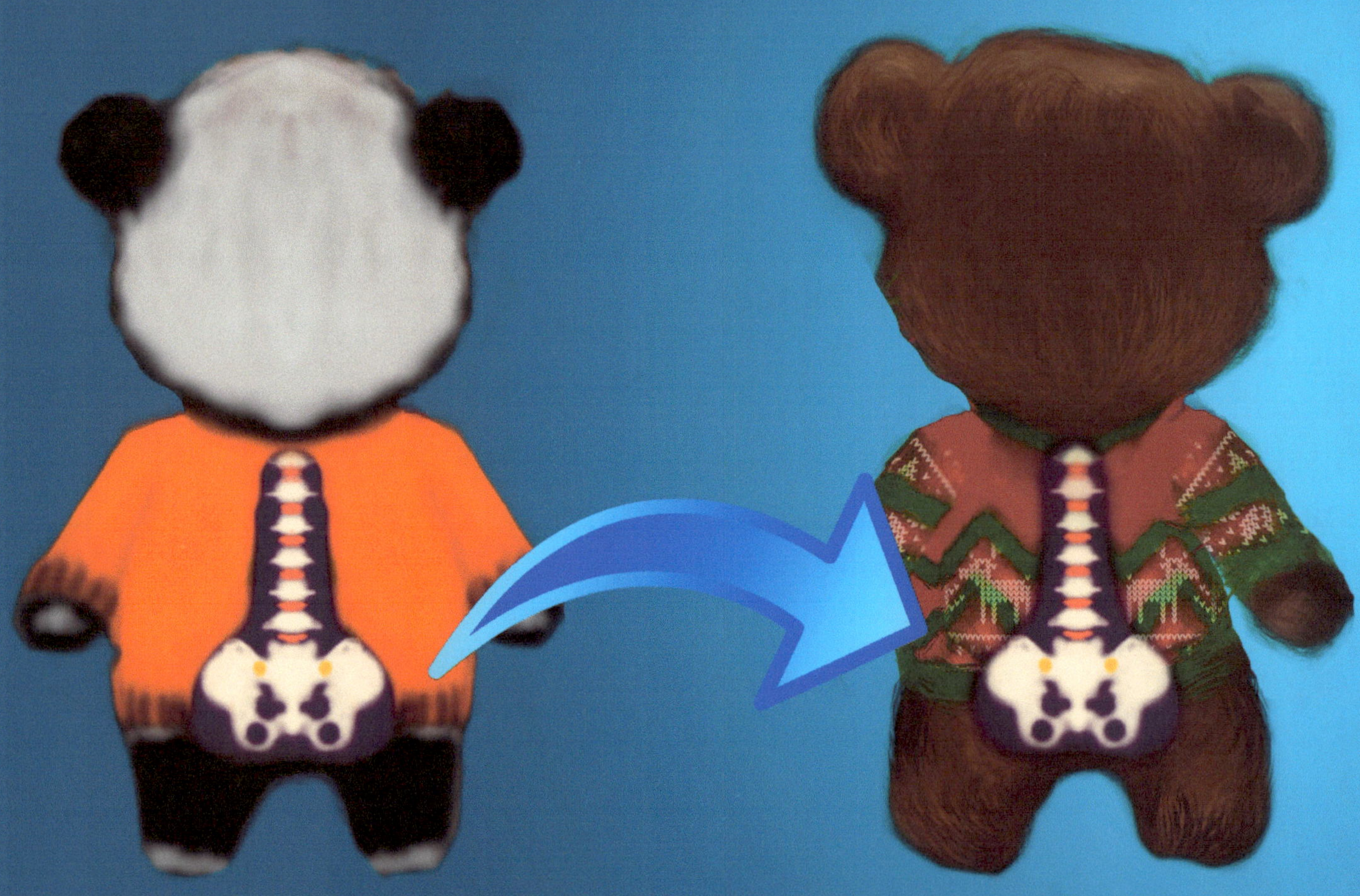

Healthy bone marrow
Sick bone marrow

"Do all people with cancer need to get a stem cell transplantation?"

"Not all. You need this treatment because your bone marrow is not working properly, but soon you'll be cured!"

"Great! But what exactly is stem cell transplantation?"

"We need to find a teddy bear with bone marrow that is just like yours. We'll use a long needle to collect some cells from the bone marrow of this teddy bear. These cells will be put inside you through a small needle in your arm. This prick will be just like that prick from yesterday."

"Will the cells from the other teddy bear's bone marrow fix mine?"

"Yes. Healthy bone marrow cells — stem cells! — are magical. When we put these cells into your arm, they'll go directly to your bone marrow!"

"How do they know where they should go?"

"It's natural. Like animals that know their way home by instinct. Medical professionals that work with stem cell transplantations use the words 'homing instinct' to explain what these cells do. Don't worry! As soon as we put the cells from your friend into your arm, they'll go to your bone marrow. That will be their new home, and they will fix it."

"What an interesting thing!"

"It's beautiful, isn't it?"

"Yes! So, Doctor, will I be cured before Christmas?"

"I think it may be possible."

"OK."

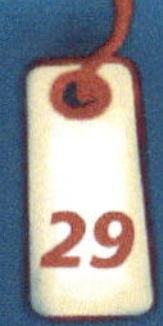

"The chemotherapy will affect your whole body, and you will lose your hair." Doctor Doll smiled. "But when the treatment is over, your cute hair will grow back!"

"Ok… Will I be able to play with my friends?"

"A teddy bear can't get cancer from other teddy bears. People either. It's not like a cold. You can play with people and teddy bears and do whatever you like! And remember that cancer is nobody's fault."

"When will I start the treatment?"

"Today. While you receive chemotherapy, we'll find a teddy bear with matching bone marrow. Then, you`ll have some rest days before you have to repeat the chemotherapy. You can play in the store on your rest days, but for now you should wait in your bed. The pharmacist will prepare the chemotherapy especially for you, and the nurse will bring it soon."

"OK. Thank you, Doctor."

The doctor went to talk with the pharmacist about Chubby. Wearing big, transparent goggles and a white coat, the pharmacist stood in a box on a nearby shelf. Just like the others, she was waiting for a kid to take her home. The doctor and her colleague, the scientist, went down to the first floor to find a teddy bear from the same lot as Chubby. They checked the teddy bears' tags. Bearnard had the same lot number as Chubby, so they asked him to help his friend. After the doctor explained all about Chubby, Bearnard was very happy to help.

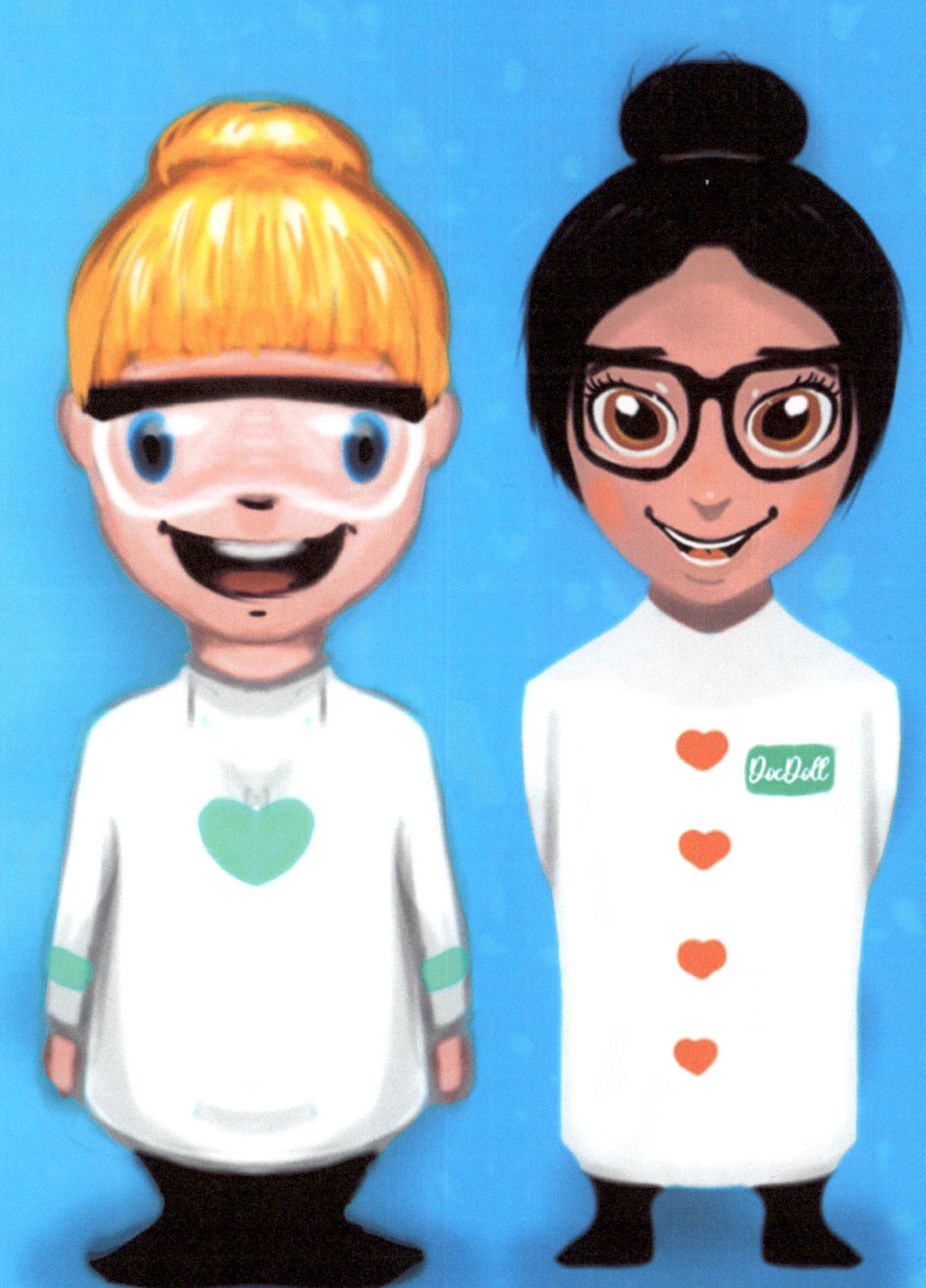
DocDoll

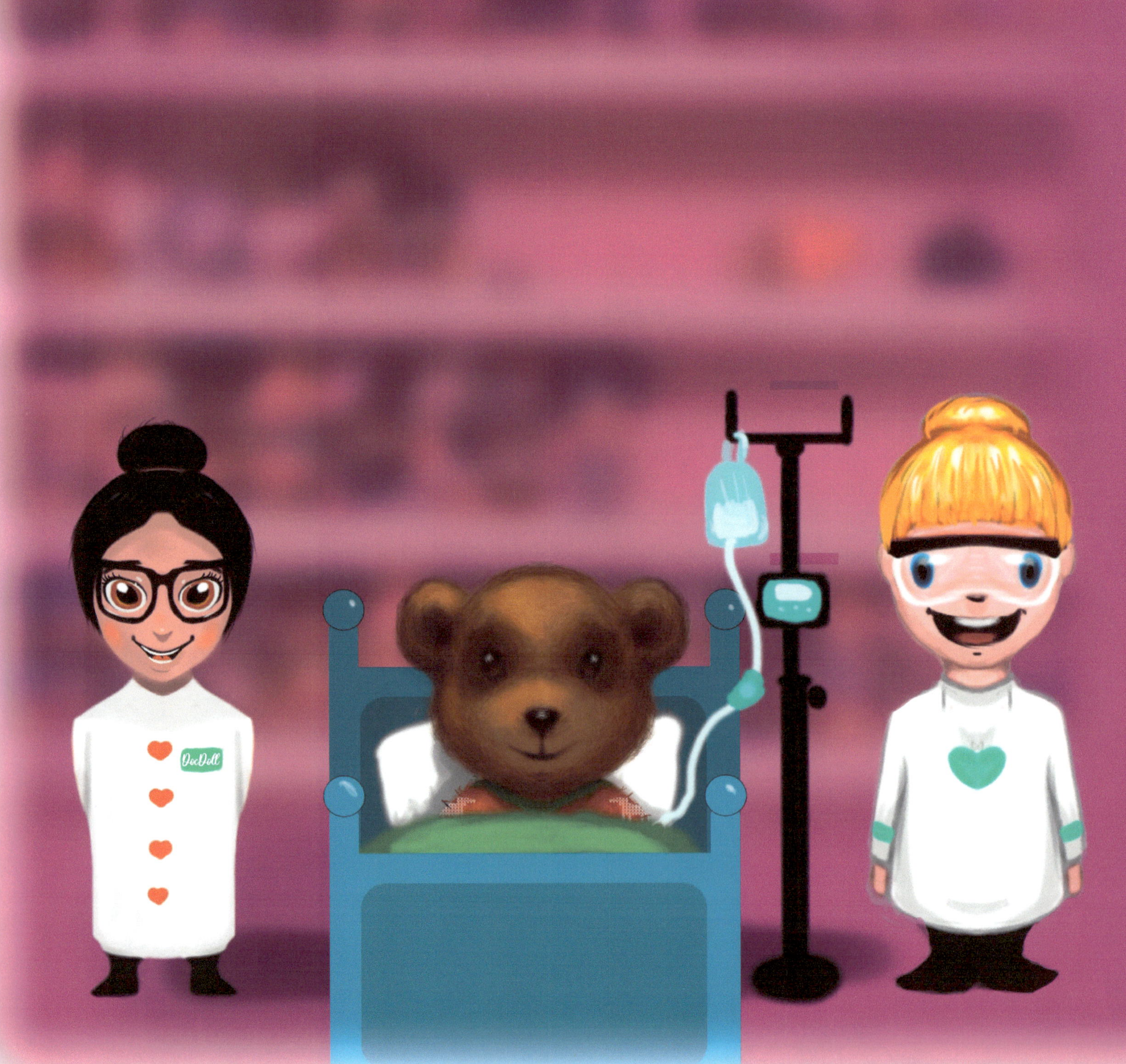
DocDoll

The pharmacist went in search of the drugs, diluents and all she needed to prepare the chemotherapy especially for Chubby. She prepared three bags, each bag with a different drug. As soon as the pharmacist had prepared the three bags of chemotherapy, the nurse picked them up and went to Chubby. The nurse used a little needle for the IV in Chubby's arm, so the drug could enter his body and eliminate the unhealthy cells.

The days passed. Chubby received chemotherapy on some days and played on the others. Finally, the big day had come. Some cells of Bearnard's bone marrow were collected, and Chubby received these stem cells through a small IV in his arm. The magical cells went to their new home and made Chubby's bone marrow healthy! On December 23rd, the doctor said, "Chubby, you are cured!"

"Thank you, Doctor. I'm a bit hairless now, but I'm happy to be cured! I'll go back to my shelf, on the first floor, to wait for a kid. I hope a kid comes soon to take me home."

"Good luck, Chubby! I'll go back to my box to wait for a kid, too." She grinned at him.

Chubby climbed into his yellow Beetle and drove to the elevator. He left the car, pressed the button in the elevator, and waited. As Chubby left the elevator, cured and honking the Beetle, his friends greeted him warmly and clapped. Chubby climbed back to the shelf and waited for the opening of the toy store.

I don't expect that a kid will take me home today. But maybe I can go home next year, when my hair has regrown. It's not that bad waiting here, after all, Chubby thought.

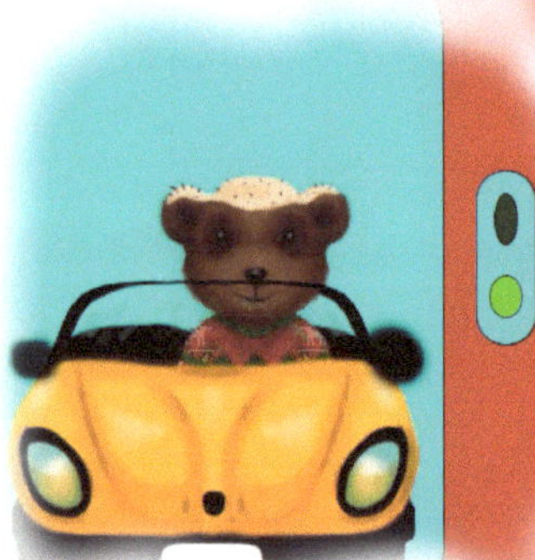

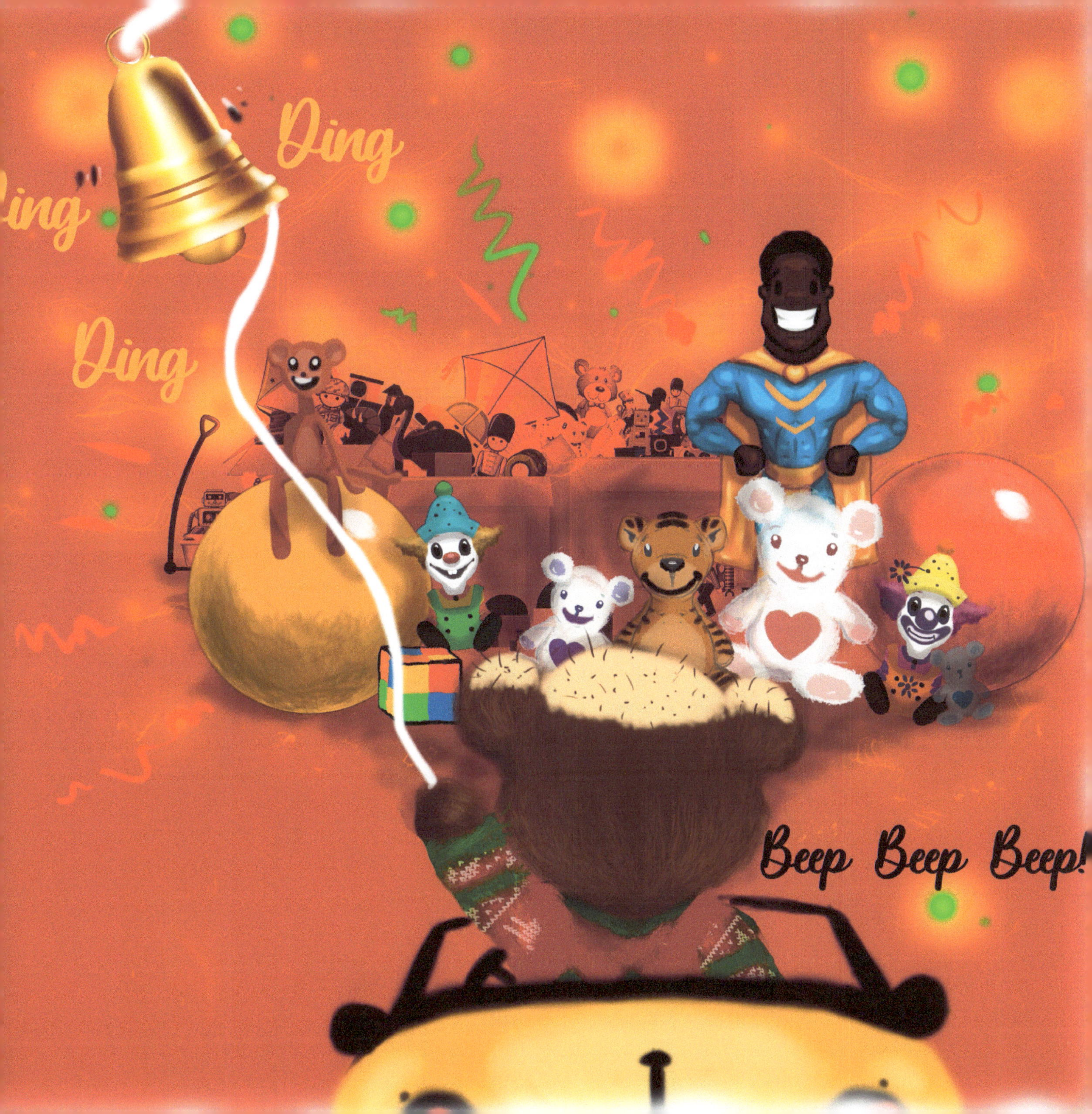
Ding
Ding
Ding
Beep Beep Beep!

On the morning of Christmas Eve, a kid named ……………………………….. (write your name on this line) entered the store.

"Mom, look how awesome this teddy bear is! He doesn't look like the others. What a style! I like him. He's so cool with that haircut! Look at the tag. His name is Chubby! Can Chubby be my Christmas present?"

"Okay, darling," said the mom.

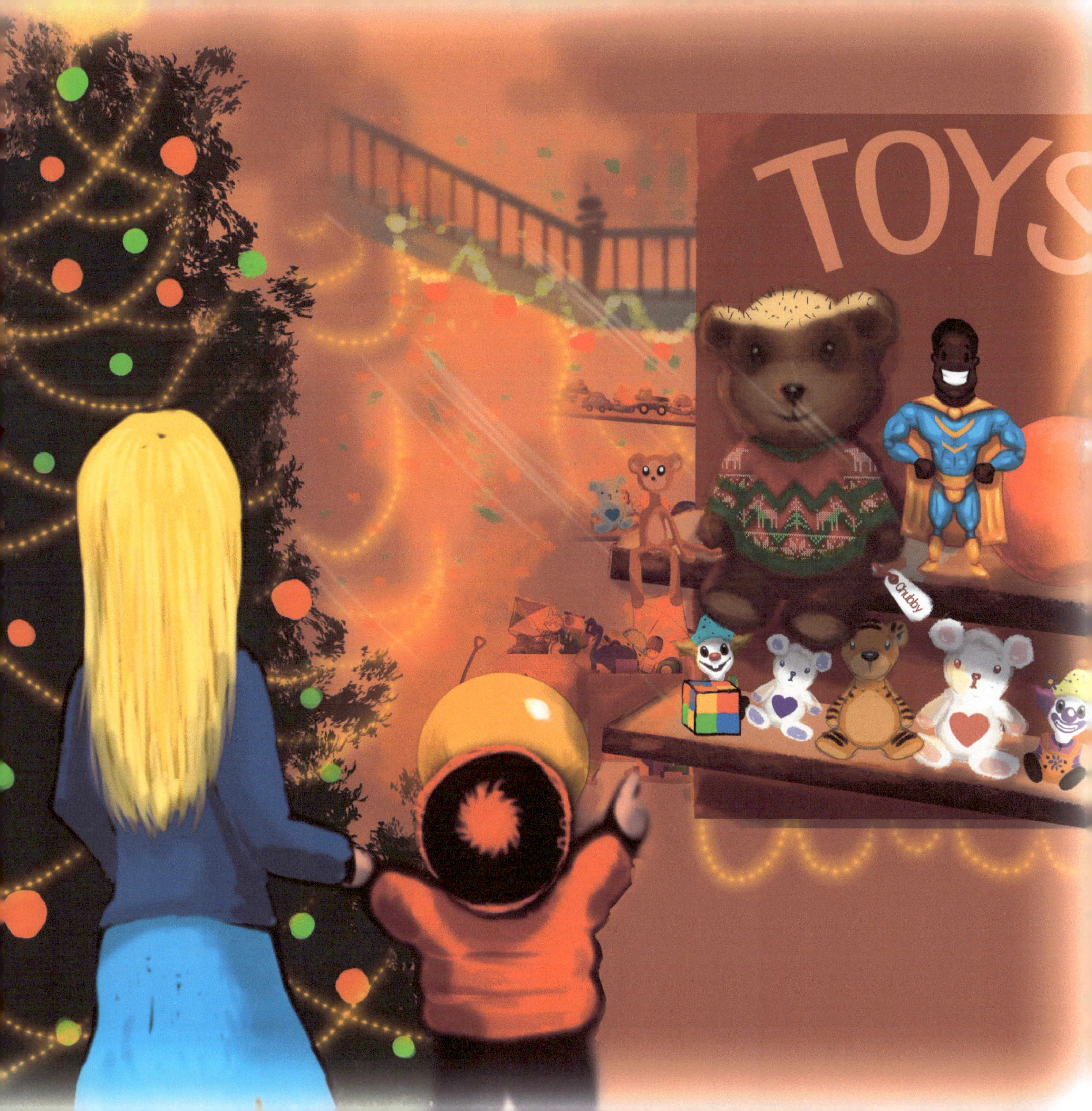
TOYS
Chubby

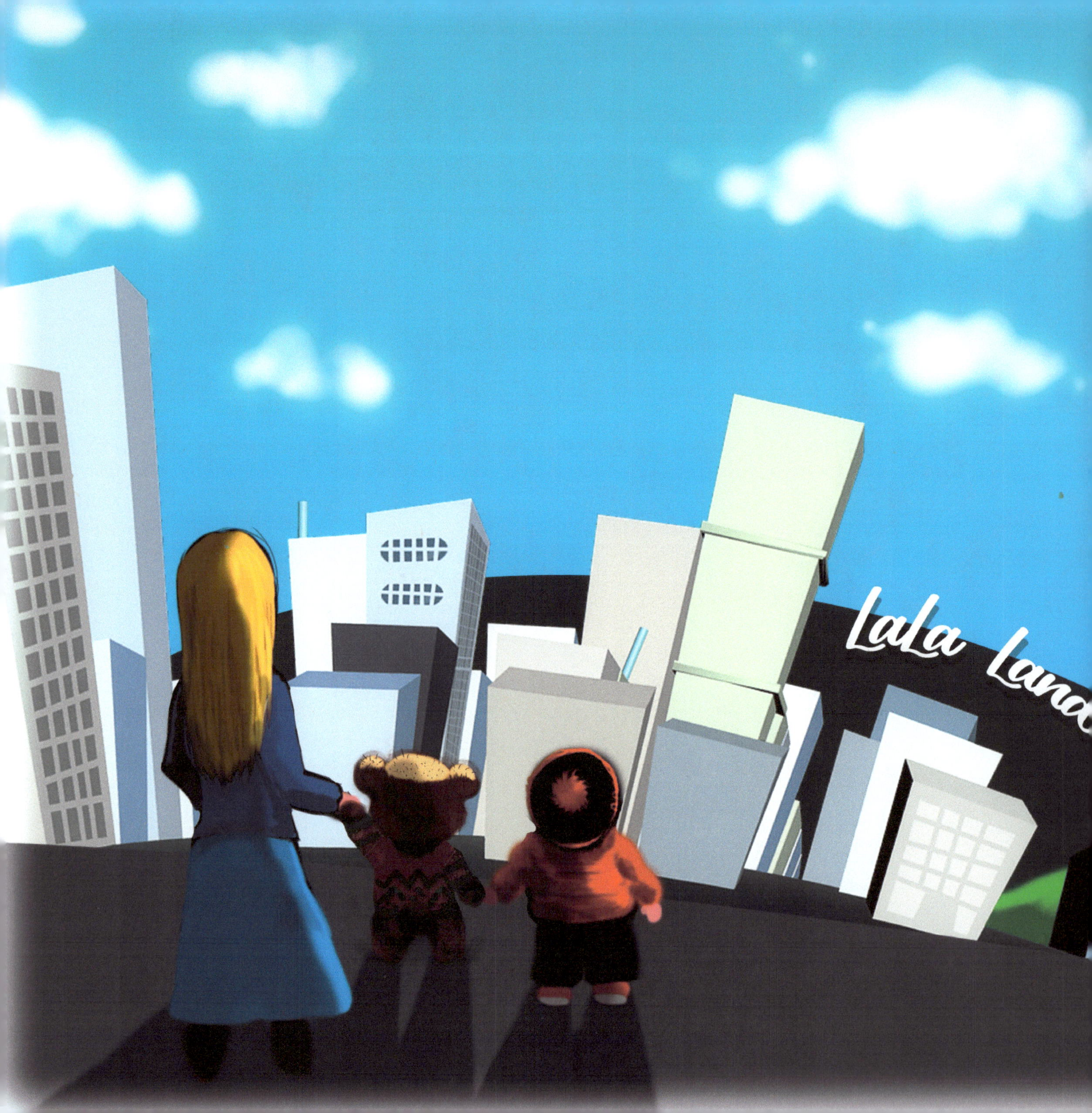

LaLa Land

The kid took Chubby's paw. Chubby held the kid's hand…
and so Chubby was taken to a real home.

When Chubby entered the coolest bedroom he ever saw,
he knew it was homing instinct that had pulled him there.

Let's Color!

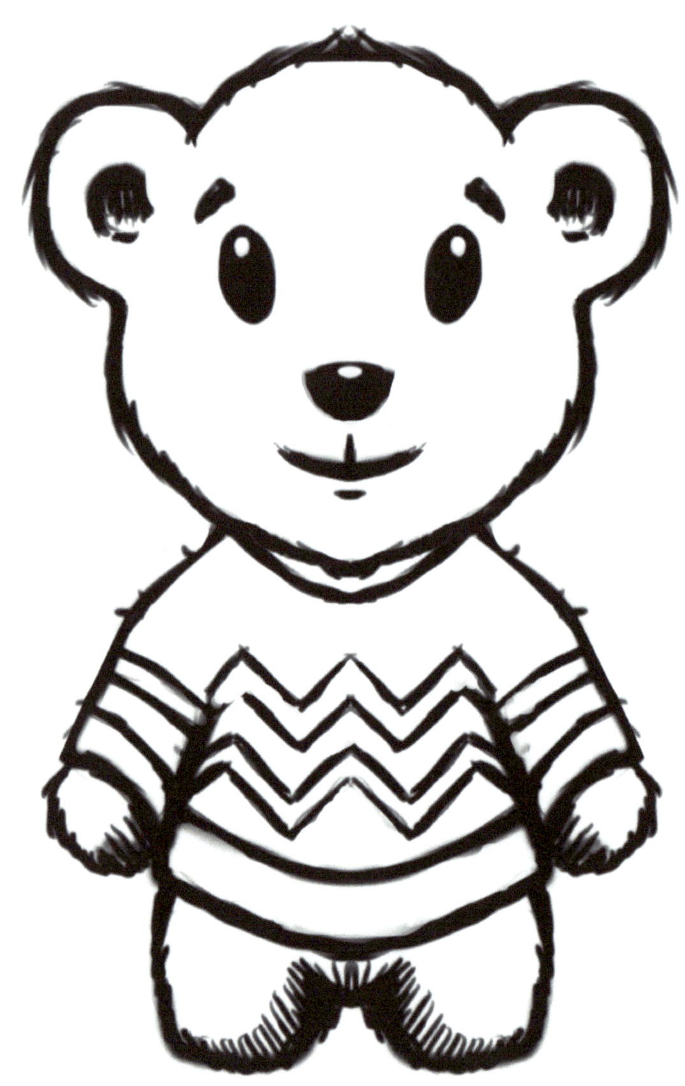

Dear Best Friend,

Now you know my story! Would you like to tell me yours?
I would love to hear it. Write your story and read it to me!

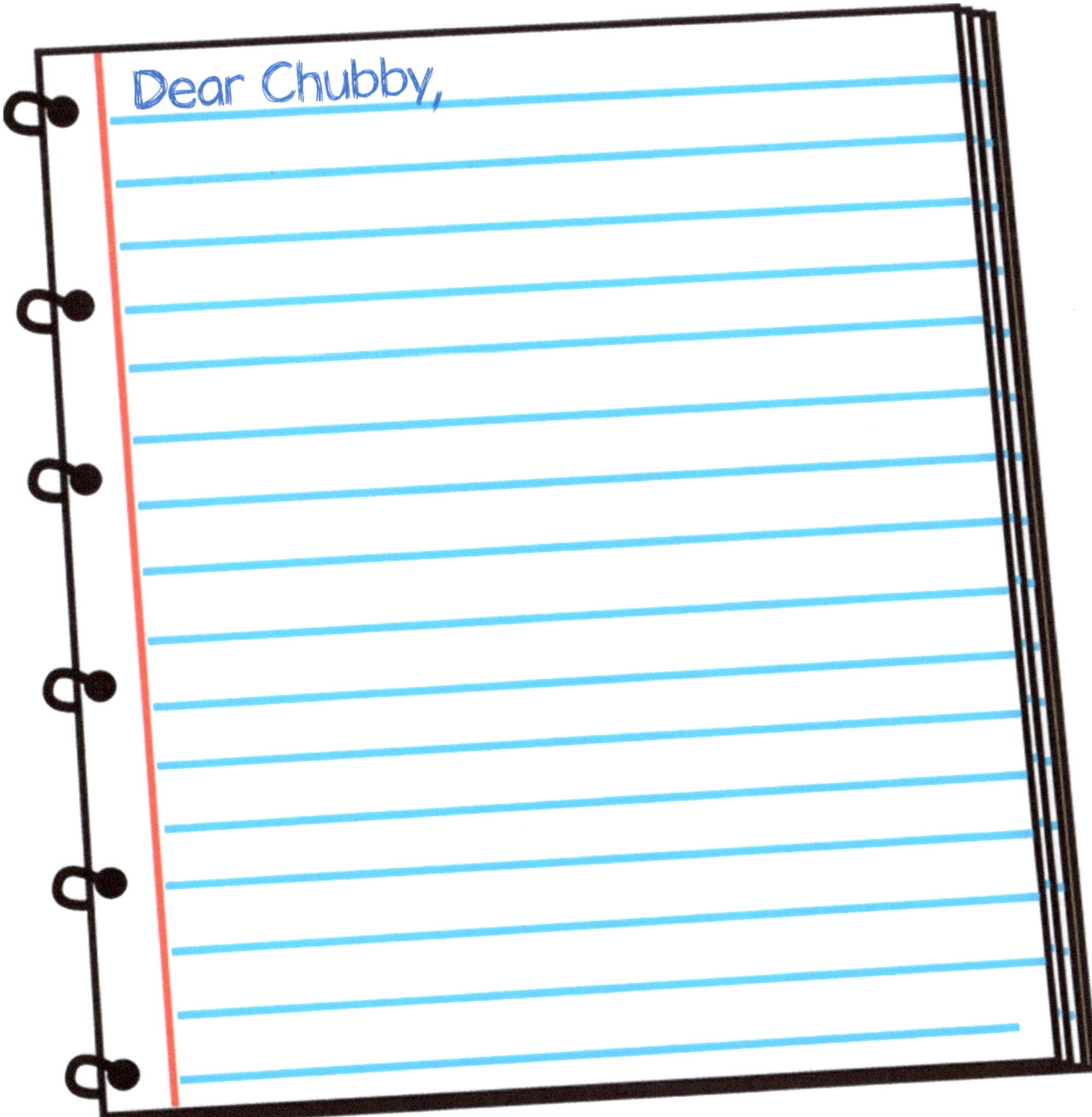

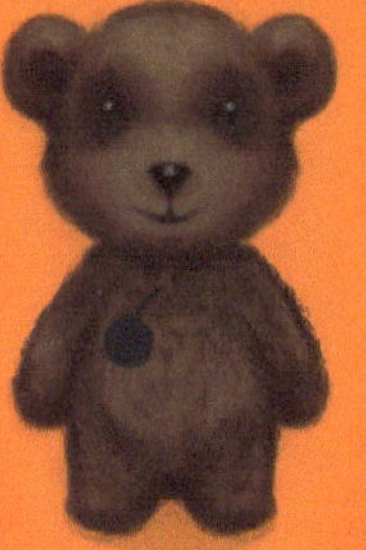

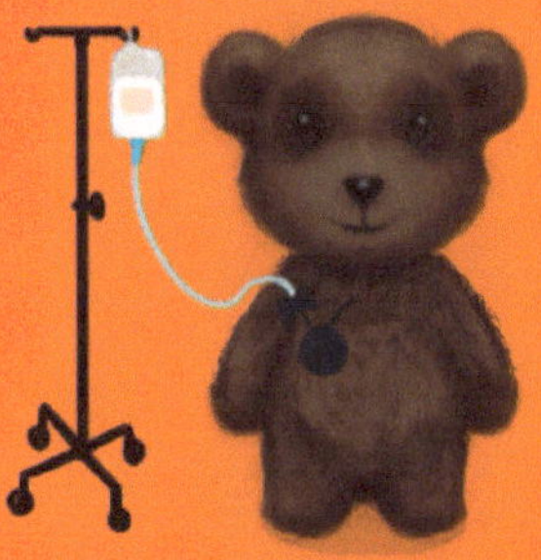

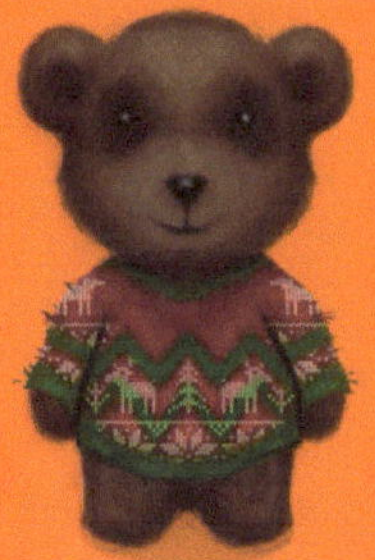

Catheter & Chemo Paper Toy

Chubby, the lovely teddy bear with a wool pullover and no pants, needs your help.

Let's insert his catheter and help him with his chemo.

Chubby is a character from the book Chubby's Tale:
The true story of a teddy bear who beat cancer (Carola Schmidt; illustrated by Vinicius Melo.)

You can print Chubby's Catheter & Chemo Paper Toy at kidscancerbooks.com

Chubby

CUT
FOLD

CHUBBY´S TALE
THE TRUE STORY OF A TEDDY BEAR
WHO BEAT CANCER

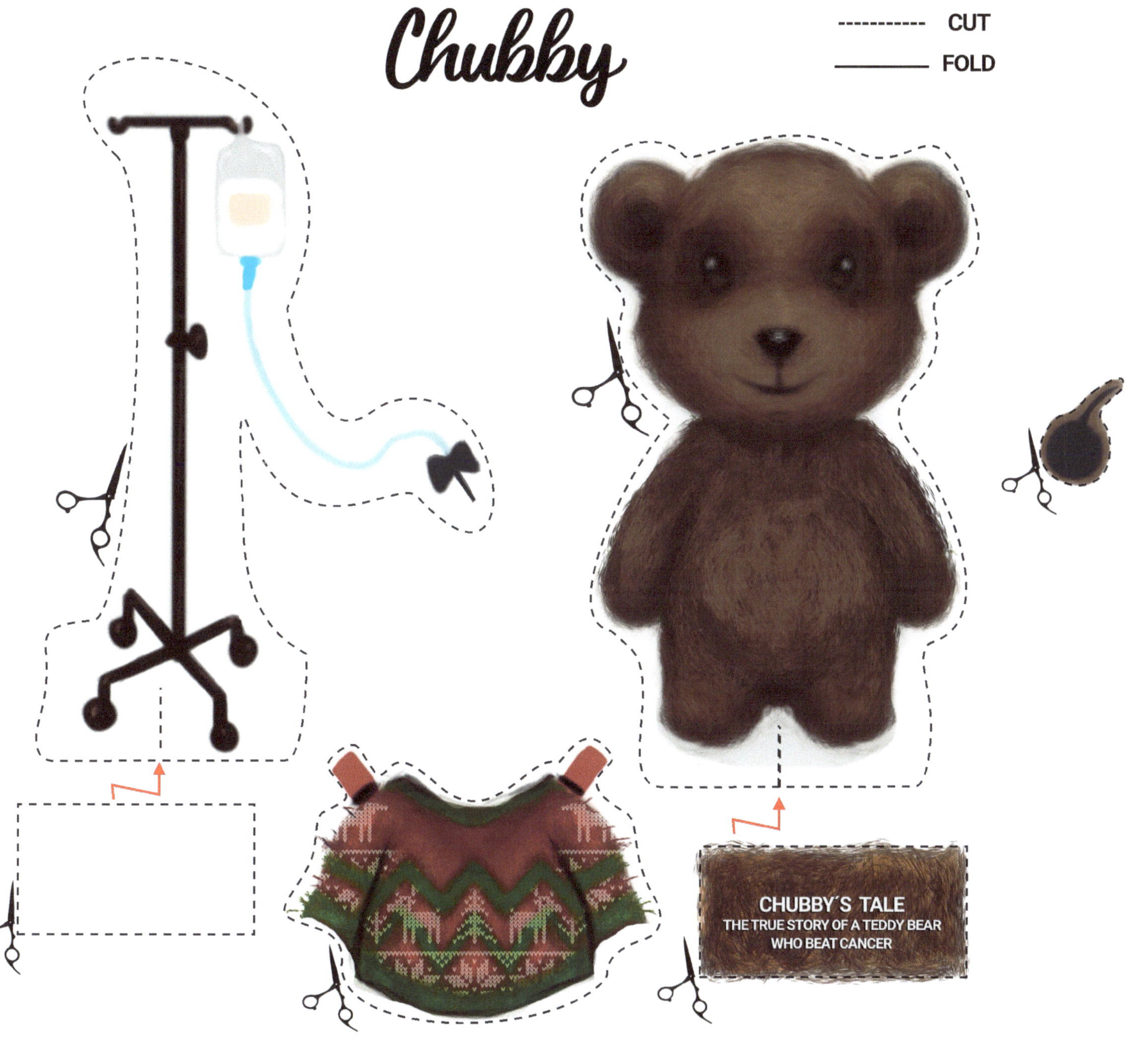

CAROLA SCHMIDT
PEDIATRIC ONCOLOGY PHARMACIST

Let's beat cancer with science and love!

CAROLA HAS EXTENSIVE EXPERIENCE IN CHEMOTHERAPY AND STEM CELL TRANSPLANTATION FOR CHILDREN AND HAS HANDLED THOUSANDS OF DOSES FOR KIDS OF ALL AGES, INCLUDING BABIES. SHE IS AN ONCOLOGICAL HOSPITAL PHARMACY SPECIALIST WITH AN MBA IN PLANNING AND BUSINESS MANAGEMENT, AND HAS EXPERIENCE WITH ADULT ONCOLOGY, AS WELL.

HER ACADEMIC STUDIES INCLUDE EXPERIENCE IN PHARMACY, PEDIATRICS, ONCOLOGY AND HEMATOLOGY, AND TEACHING AT THE PEDIATRIC ONCOLOGY HEMATOLOGY PROGRAM IN THE BIGGEST PEDIATRIC HOSPITAL IN BRAZIL. AFTER COLLEGE SHE GAINED A WEALTH OF EXPERIENCE AT HOSPITALS, CLINICS, AND PHARMACIES, WORKING WITH DRUG INTERACTIONS, PEDIATRICS, ONCOLOGY, HEMATOLOGY, STEM CELL TRANSPLANTATION, NEONATOLOGY, INTENSIVE HEALTH CARE AND INFECTOLOGY. CAROLA HAS THE EXPERIENCE OF WORKING IN HUGE MEDICAL CENTERS IN BRAZIL, SOME OF THEM WITHOUT RESOURCES, DEMANDING A LOT OF CREATIVITY, RESEARCH AND KNOWLEDGE. HER RESEARCH AND TREATMENTS ARE USED IN THE VERY BEST HOSPITALS, AND SHE CONTINUES TO DEVELOP AND PUBLISH GUIDELINES TO HELP HEALTHCARE PROFESSIONALS WORLDWIDE.

"BELONGING" IS A SUBJECT THAT HAS ALWAYS FASCINATED HER AND DIRECTS HER WRITING FOR CHILDREN'S BOOKS. SHE BELIEVES THAT EACH OF US HAS OUR OWN STORIES, HISTORY AND THE DESIRE TO BELONG. HER FAVORITE WORD IS "HOMING." WHEN SHE LEARNED ABOUT HOMING OF STEM CELLS, SHE FELL IN LOVE WITH THE COMPLEX BIOCHEMICAL PROCESSES THAT MAKE STEM CELLS (THAT ARE COLLECTED FROM A DONOR'S BONE MARROW) ABLE TO BE INFUSED INTO A RECEPTOR'S ARM VEIN—THEY CAN FIND THEIR WAY HOME TO THE RECEPTOR'S BONE MARROW! HOMING, FOR HER, IS HIGHLY RELATED TO BELONGING. THESE THEMES GAVE HER THE IDEA TO WRITE CHUBBY'S TALE: THE TRUE STORY OF A TEDDY BEAR WHO BEAT CANCER. SHE IS THE AUTHOR OF SEVERAL SCIENTIFIC BOOKS IN PEDIATRIC ONCOLOGY PUBLISHED BY SPRINGER NATURE.

KIDSCANCERBOOKS.COM

ALSO BY CAROLA SCHMIDT

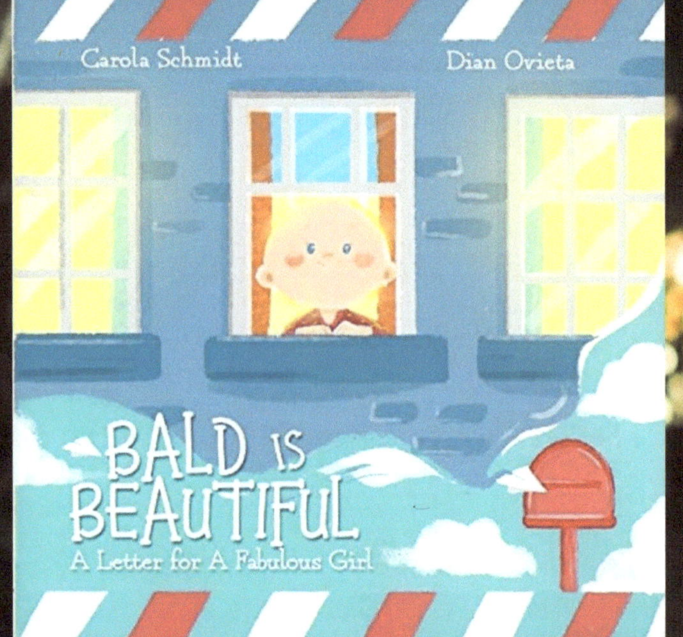

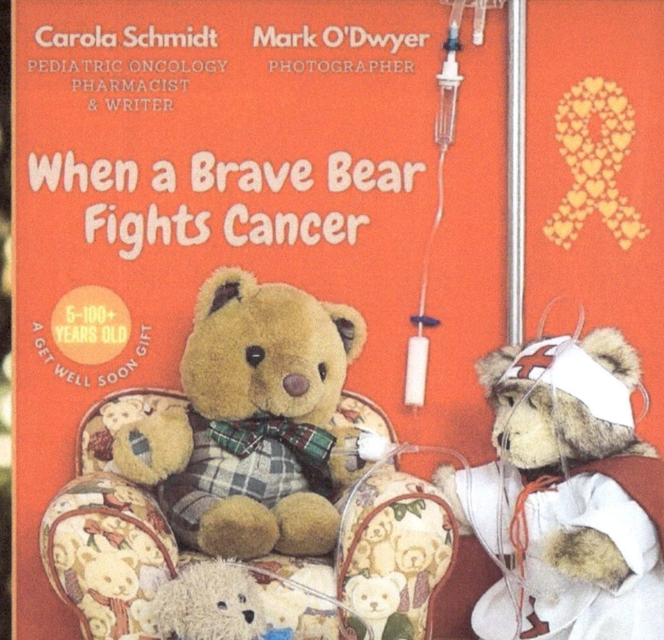

KIDSCANCERBOOKS.COM

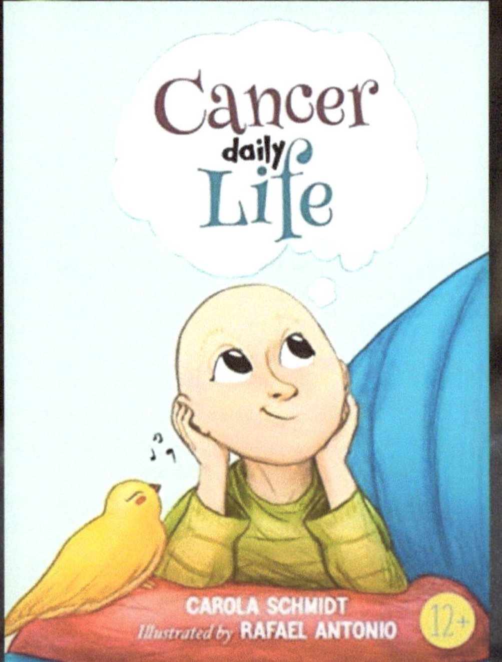

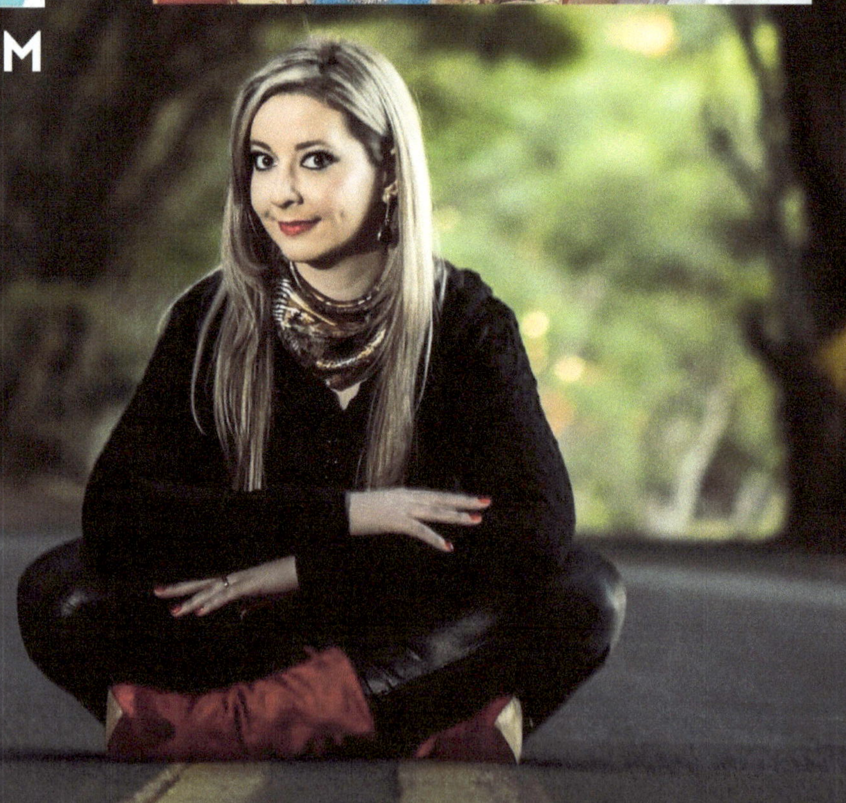